ATHEROSCLEROSIS: UNDERSTANDING PATHOGENESIS AND CHALLENGE FOR TREATMENT

ATHEROSCLEROSIS: UNDERSTANDING PATHOGENESIS AND CHALLENGE FOR TREATMENT

SLAVICA MITROVSKA
SILVANA JOVANOVA
INGE MATTHIESEN
AND
CHRISTIAN LIBERMANS

Nova Biomedical Books
New York

For permission to use material from this book please contact us:
Telephone 631-231-7269; Fax 631-231-8175
Web Site: http://www.novapublishers.com

Library of Congress Cataloging-in-Publication Data

ISBN: 978-1-60692-677-2

Available upon request

Published by Nova Science Publishers, Inc. ✝ New York

Contents

Preface

Atherosclerosis is a chronic inflammatory disease that affects medium and large-sized arteries. It begins after birth and the progression depends on several factors – traditional triad: hypertension, hyperlipidemia and diabetes mellitus, then age, sex, smoking and sedentary life-style. At the beginning atherosclerosis is asymptomatic and we cannot estimate appropriately its frequency, but its complications – coronary artery diseases, cerebrovascular diseases, peripheral arterial diseases, which occur late, are responsible for more than half of the yearly mortality in the world. Unfortunately, sudden cardiac death may be the first clinical manifestation.

The incipient event is endothelial dysfunction, as a result of injury, caused by high level of cholesterol [especially low-density-lipoprotein LDL], hyperglycemia, hypertension, smoking, infectious agents, and toxins. Endothelial cells overexpress adhesion molecules – vascular cell adhesion molecule–1 [VCAM-1] and increases recruitment of inflammatory cells– monocytes [Mo], T-cells and subsequent release of monocyte chemo–attractant protein–1 [MCP-1] that results in additional leucocytes recruitment. Injured endothelium allows migration of inflammatory cells that release cytokines and lipids into the intima. That leads to cytokine-mediated progression of atherosclerosis and oxidation of LDL. Macrophages [MP] take up oxi-LDL and form foam-cell. They have metabolic activity and produce cytokines, proliferation of smooth muscle cells and formulate athero-fibrose plaque. Atherosclerotic plaque is composed of superficial layer – fibrose cap and lipid core, that consists of foam cells, extracellular lipid and necrotic cellular debris. It progresses as a result of accumulation of lipid and proliferation of smooth muscle cells and results in luminal narrowing of the arteries which leads to compromised blood and oxygen supply to the tissues. The gradually growing atherosclerotic plaques have thick fibrose cap and are stable. They cause symptoms of stable angina. Rapidly growing plaques cause unstable coronary artery disease. These plaques are mainly composed of lipids and have tiny fibrose cap that is prone to fissuring or rupture. Intraplaque hemorrhage from microvessels in plaque initiate platelet adhesion and activation of coagulation cascade that leads to platelet thrombus formation, i.e. promote thrombogenesis.

Knowledge of the pathogenesis of the atherothrombosis modifies the diagnostic and therapeutic approach.

Conclusion: Our attention should be focused on the management of three points:

1. Endothelial dysfunction [correction of modified risk factors: hypertension, hyperlipidemia, diabetes mellitus, life-style-smoking, physical activity and food],
2. Atherosclerosis [modification of the inflammatory cascade, i.e. elimination of inflammatory pathways and inhibition of oxidation of LDL],
3. Thrombogenesis [inhibition of platelet adhesion, activation and aggregation].

Keywords: *atherosclerosis, endothelial dysfunction, inflammatory pathways, thrombogenesis.*

Chapter I

Introduction

Atherosclerosis is a chronic inflammatory disease that affects medium and large-sized arteries. It begins after birth, initially it is a silent process but it progresses during the person's life. The atherosclerotic lesions are a result of continuum molecular and cellular interaction between vessel wall and blood constituents, release of number of signaling pathways and activation of the inflammatory and coagulation cascades that lead to structural changes. At the beginning atherosclerosis is asymptomatic and we cannot estimate appropriately its frequency. But, in some people atherosclerosis has rapid progress and triggers a vicious circle that leads to clinical manifestations of coronary artery diseases, cerebrovascular diseases, and peripheral arterial diseases. Unfortunately, sudden cardiac death may be the first clinical manifestation. The increasing incidence makes the atherosclerosis a leader of morbidity and mortality in the developing world.

According to the American Heart Association, more than 11 million people suffer from coronary artery disease [CAD] in USA, 30% have carotid artery disease, 1.5 million myocardial infarctions per year, more than 200,000 deaths per year caused by cerebrovascular diseases [1].

The other thing that should be a concern is the increasingly younger age group having onset of symptoms, as early as 35 years old. The progress of atherosclerosis depends on several factors – traditional triad: hypertension, hyperlipidemia and diabetes mellitus, than age, sex, stress, smoking and sedentary life-style [2].

Chapter II

Impaired Endothelial Function

The incipient changes occur in the endothelium and the earliest step is impaired endothelial function. Endothelium is an inner layer of the vessel wall that has an active role to respond to various stimuli. It acts as an endocrine organ that has secretory role and it takes place in the process of inflammation, hemostasis and fibroproliferative process. Also, endothelium regulates the vessel wall tonus by release endothelium derived relaxing [EDRF] and constrictive factors. The vasodilatation is providing by EDRF – nitric oxide [NO], produced by NO synthase enzyme [type III eNOS], whereas vasoconstriction is mediated by endothelin-1 [ET-1] and thromboxane A_2. The imbalance between vasodilatative and vasoconstrictive substances leads to the impairment of endothelial cell function. This is the first stage of atherosclerotic process – lack of activity of endothelium derived NO and impaired vascular relaxation. In the setting of hypertension, hyperlipidemia [especially high level of LDL-C], diabetes mellitus, genetic alterations, smoking, toxins, infectious agents, the blood flow became turbulent and provoked a number of insults to the endothelium [3].

Chapter III

Inflammatory Pathways Promote Atherosclerosis

As a "response to injury" the endothelium becomes active and initiates a cascade of subsequent events, which are compensatory mechanisms to keep the homeostasis. If the influence of provocative agents continues excessively, than these mechanisms overdrive normal properties of the endothelium and lead to the development of atherosclerotic plaque. The activated endothelium over expresses adhesion molecules, as vascular cell adhesion molecule-1 [VCAM-1] and increases recruitment of inflammatory cells - monocytes [Mo], T-cells and subsequent release of monocytchemo-attractant protein-1 [MCP-1] that results in their differentiation into macrophages [MP] [4].

In the acute phase, the inflammatory cells secrete a number of cytokines, mostly interleukins – IL-1ß, IL-6, IL-8, than tumor necrosis factor- α [TNF-α], interferon-γ [IFN-γ] and transforming growth factor-ß [TFG-ß] [5]. They increase permeability of the endothelium to lipoproteins, especially low-density-lipoproteins [LDL-C] and they have enhanced migration through the endothelial membrane into subendothelium. LDL deposit initiates additional induction of numbers MP and release of cytokines [especially IL-1], hydrolytic enzymes and chemokines, growth factors and a vicious circle of inflammation starts [6]. Increased accumulation of MP is associated with increased level of fibrogen and C-reactive protein [CRP]. It is believed that CRP helps the MP in the process of phagocytosis.

Intra intimal LDL undergoes oxidation [oxidant stress] by oxidant mechanisms that involve hydrogen peroxide and free radicals. MP recognizes and phagocyte oxidized low-density-lipoproteins [oxi-LDL] through scavenger receptors [7]. Accumulation of oxi-LDL and cholesterol esters in MP leads to formation of foam cells. Oxidized LDL have toxic effects. They produce free radicals that reduce activity of NO-synthase and inactivation of NO leads to vasoconstriction [8].

The foam cells have metabolic activity, secrete TGF-ß, stimulating the proliferation of smooth muscle cells, fibroblasts, collagen and elastin and form fibrous cap over the lipid collection. Thus, the atherofibrous plaque is formed [9].

Chapter IV

The Composition of the Atherosclerotic Plaque

Atherosclerotic plaque progresses as a result of the progressive accumulation of lipids and proliferation of smooth muscle cells. As long as injurious agents persist, the affected endothelium reacts with abnormal inflammatory and fibroproliferative response, triggering the progression of atherosclerotic plaque, as well as the disease progression. Development of plaque deforms the arterial wall.

The gradually growing plaques cause thickening of the artery wall. The arterial wall becomes rigid. At the beginning they do not compromise arterial circulation. These plaques are angiographically invisible and according to the American Heart Association, are classified as type IV and V-a [10]. At that stage, the lumen of the artery remains unaltered due to "remodeling," compensatory dilatation of the wall, termed – Glagov phenomenon. Further enlargement of the lesion results in luminal narrowing and compromising of the blood and oxygen supply [11].

The gradually growing atherosclerotic plaques have a thick fibrous cap. They are stable and when the narrowing of the lumen is more than 50%, cause the symptoms of chronic stable angina. Clinicians note that these patients have better prognosis despite critical diminution of the coronary artery flow. Contrary, potentially dangerous lesions are usually nonocclusive. Thus, retrospective analyses of angiographic observations revealed that almost 2/3 of patients with acute coronary syndromes [unstable angina and myocardial infarction] have low-grade stenosis less than 70% [mostly < 50%]. Morphologic examinations have shown that these plaques are composed mainly of lipids and have a tiny fibrous cap [12].

These findings lead our attention to the other direction, to the composition of the atherosclerotic plaque, as an important predictor of adverse cardiac events.

In 1992, James Muller introduces the term "vulnerable" plaque. It is a morphologic description and concerns the cellular and molecular characteristics of the atherosclerotic plaques that are prone to rupture [13].

Peter Libby et al. describe vulnerable plaque as a lesion consisting of a central lipid-rich core, surrounded by a tiny fibrous cap [14]. Davies et al. estimate that the lipid core is 30-40% of the vulnerable plaque volume [15].

Lipid-rich core is composed of lipid-laden foam cells, necrotic cellular debris, extracellular lipid, free and esterified cholesterol and cholesterol esters.

The thickness of the fibrous cap is a second condition for stability/instability of the plaque. The tiny cap is collagen-deficient and also contains less proteoglicans. These things make the cap much more susceptible to destroying enzymes – matrix metalloproteinase (MMPs) that include collagenase and gelatinase and prone to disruption. Burne et al. define the fibrous cap as vulnerable if its thickness is less than 65 μm [16].

Several results from coronary atherectomy have shown that the culprit lesion in patients with unstable angina has increased neovascularization. These vasa vasorum that proliferate within the plaque are fragile and cause intraplaque hemorrhage with secondary rupture [17].

Concerning the mechanism of instability of atherosclerotic plaque, most of the theories accentuate the imbalance between presences of normal and inflammatory cells [18]. Thus, inflammatory cells, especially T-Ly, have a tendency to localize in the "shoulders" of the plaque. These sites are lesion prone sites. T-Ly produce cytokine, CD40 ligand, IFN-γ that impairs collagen synthesis and IL-1β and IL-4 stimulate MP to produce MMP that degrade the fibrous cap. The result of this activity is plaque rupture or plaque erosion and exposition of thrombogenic substances of the core to the blood [19].

Chapter V

Thrombogenesis

Normal endothelium maintains the platelets in a resting state by producing prostacyclin and NO. Loss of endothelium exposes the subendothelium to the blood constituents and initiates the activation of coagulation cascade [20]. Thus, the procoagulant milieu favors thrombus formation. The subendothelium releases von Willebrand factor and other adhesive proteins that bind to glycoprotein receptor Ib [GP Ib] on the platelet surface and provoke platelet adhesion to the subendothelial collagen. Furthermore, adhered platelets became active, secrete adenosine-diphosphate [ADP] and number of mediators-cytokines, Thrombocyte derived growth factor, Thrombocyte factor-4, C-reactive protein, TGF- β, Placental growth factor [PlGF] and together with thrombin promote platelet aggregation [21].

Final step in the process of thrombogenesis is the activation of the GP IIb/IIIa receptors of the platelet surface, and together with fibrinogen make tight connection between platelets. That leads to thrombus formation [22]. This is a defensive mechanism, to protect the organism from bleeding. Activation of platelets involves triggering of internal signaling pathways, as a releasing of adenosine diphosphate [ADP], serotonin, calcium and recruitment of more platelets. But sometimes those triggers became uncontrolled and thrombus formation culminates in thrombosis. The final outcome is occlusion of the artery and consecutive events – stable, unstable angina or myocardial infarction.

Thus thrombogenesis has become the second most important process in pathogenesis of acute coronary syndrome [23].

Chapter VI

Therapeutic Approaches

The base of human physiology is to keep the balance between restoring and destroying processes. For this purpose, each process in the human body consists of pro and contra mechanisms [proinflammatory and anti-inflammatory, procoagulant and anticoagulant elements]. The aim is to maintain the equilibrium and to provide normal function for each organ.

The nature of the processes of atherosclerosis and thrombogenesis, as well as their alterations and signaling pathways, are a challenge for observation and action [24].

Considering that atherosclerosis begins at birth and progresses during one's lifetime, maybe we should accept it as a part of biologic evolution, as a part of the natural aging process. The question is why, what and when this process became out of control? Why some people develop rapid process of atherosclerosis? What are the provocative factors that trigger uncontrolled inflammatory, prothrombotic and fibroproliferative signaling pathways[25]?

Exploring these reasons, we review the current therapeutic modalities. Thus, the mechanical revascularization techniques [angiography/stenting as well as by-pass surgery] are palliative treatments. They have excellent results in reducing the incidence of adverse cardiac events (recurrent angina, myocardial [re]infarction, heart failure, cerebrovascular insult, death), but these are a secondary prevention. The process of atherosclerosis continues [in-stent restenosis, graft stenosis]. So, we need to focus on primary prevention. Peter Libby suggests, "the concept of interventional cardiology must expand beyond mechanical revascularization to encompass preventive interventions that forestall future events" [26].

In this regard we need to focus our attention in three directions:

1. Correction of the established risk factors: [control the blood pressure, hyperlipidemia, diabetes mellitus, lifestyle modification, smoking, physical activity and food],
2. Modification of the inflammatory cascade, i.e. elimination of inflammatory pathways and inhibition of oxidation of LDL. To enter deep into mechanisms of inflammation and address oxidative stress as a root cause,
3. Inhibition of platelet adhesion, activation and aggregation.

Chapter VII

Treatment of the Established Risk Factors

Treating casual factors (hypertension, diabetes mellitus and hyperlipidemia) is the most helpful means to control and modify the disease's progress. Smith S. and colleagues states "aggressive risk factors management improves survival, reduces recurrent events and the need for interventional procedures and improves quality of life for patients with atherosclerotic vascular disease" [27].

Hypertension provokes endothelial dysfunction and accelerates atherosclerosis. Angiotensin II, the enzyme that is elevated in patients with hypertension, causes vasoconstriction. Diminishing the concentration of this enzyme with ACE inhibitors, prevents stimulation of smooth muscle cell and inhibition of myointimal proliferation.

Also, ACE inhibitors inhibit the breakdown of bradykinin, stimulant of nitric oxide release and promote a vasodilatory effect. Their antiproliferative, anti-inflammatory and vasodilatory effects modulate atherosclerotic process [28,29].

The advanced glycosylation end products, in patients with diabetes mellitus, change the phenotype characteristics of endothelial cells. They increase adhesion of Mo on their surfaces and increase the adhesion of platelets their activation and aggregation. Patients with insulin resistance have high level of markers of inflammation (CRP), haemostasis (coagulation factors VII–IX, von Willebrand factor) and marker of endothelial dysfunction (tissue plasminogen activator [t-PA] antigens). Good glycemic control (introducing the insulin) will interfere with decreasing the inflammation, controlling the atherosclerotic lesions and thrombus formation [30].

Lifestyle modification (especially in regards to fatty food, smoking, sedentary lifestyle) contribute significantly to keep control of atherosclerosis.

Currently, the main focus is to reduce oxidative stress, oxidative damage to the endothelial cells as a base of inflammation and development of atherosclerosis. Advances in the understanding of molecular basis of atherosclerosis have shown that inflammatory pathways are included in each step of atherogenesis. Addressing the oxi-LDL, as a very active and having a toxic effect on endothelium, can slow the atherosclerotic progression. In many studies, early institution of statins, 3-hydroxy-3-metylgluteryl coenzyme A [HMG-CoA] reductase inhibitors, have shown a significant anti-inflammatory effect [31].

They have an important role in the treatment of atherosclerosis, increasing the concentrations of anti-inflammatory cytokines [IL-10] and decreasing the concentrations of proinflammatory cytokines [IL-1 and CRP]. In this way, statins have made an important contribution in reducing the consequences of atherosclerosis as well as overall mortality [32].

As thrombogenesis is a part of atherosclerotic disease, the inhibition of platelet activation and thrombin generation also contributes to improve clinical outcomes.

The analyses of several studies underlie potential benefits of inhibitors of adenosine-di-phosphate (Clopidrogrel, Ticlopidine) and inhibitors of GP IIb/IIIa receptors (Abciximab, Eptifibatide, Aggrastat) in reducing the risk of death in patients with ischemic heart disease and atherosclerosis [33, 34].

Conclusion

Atherosclerosis is an ongoing problem in modern society. Many factors that are established as risk factors for atherogenesis cause activation of the cells and signaling pathways involve in the process of inflammation. Despite many studies that offer potentionally valuable information in this regard, we still need to enter deep into pathogenesis of inflammation and search for trigger mechanisms. Understanding the pathogenesis of atherosclerosis will contribute to introduce more effective novel therapies that may modulate the course of atherosclerosis.

References

[1] American Heart Association. Heart and Stroke Facts. AHA 1996 Supplement. Dallas, TX, 1996:1-23

[2] World Health Statistics Annual, 1994. Geneva, Switzerland: World Health Organization. 1995

[3] Kinlay S, Ganz P: Relation between endothelial dysfunction and the acute coronary syndrome: implication for therapy. *Am. J. Cardiol.* 2000; 86:10J-13J

[4] Moustapha A, Anderson V: Contemporary View of The Acute Coronary Syndromes. *J. Invasive Cardiol.* 2003; 15[2]: 71-79.

[5] Ohji T, Urano H, Shirahata A et al: Transforming growth factor beta 1 and beta 2 induce down regulation of thrombomodulin in human umbilical vein endothelial cells. *Thromb. Haemost.* 1995; 73:812-818

[6] Rajavashisth TB, Liao JK, Galis ZS, et al: Inflammatory cytokines and oxidized low-density lipoproteins increase endothelial cell expression of membrane type 1-matrix metalloproteinase. *J. Biol. Chem.* 1999; 274: 11924-11929.

[7] Vieira O, et al: Oxidized LDLs alter the activity of the ubiquitin-proteasome pathway: Potential role in oxidized LDL-induces apoptosis, *Faseb. J.* 2000;14:532-542

[8] Weinbrenner T, Cladellas M, Isabel Covas M et al: High oxidative stress in patients with stable coronary heart disease. *Atherosclerosis.* 2003; 168 [1]: 99-106

[9] Galis ZS, Sukhova GK, Kranzhofer R, et al: Macrophage foam cells from experimental atheroma constitutively produce matrix-degrading proteinases. *Proc. Natl .Acad .Sci .USA* 1995; 92:402-406.

[10] Stary HC, Chandler AB, Dinsmore RE, Fuster V, Glagov S, Insull WJr, Rosenfeld ME Schwartz CJ, Wagner WD, Wissler RW: A definition of advanced types of atherosclerotic lesions and a histological classification of atherosclerosis. A report from the Commitee on Vascular Lesions of the Council on Atherosclerosis. American Heart Association. *Circulation* 1995; 92:1355-1374.

[11] Davies MJ: A macro and micro view of coronary vascular insult in ischemic heart disease. *Circulation* 1990;82 [suppl II]: II-38-II46.

[12] Stary HC: Natural history and histological classification of atherosclerotic lesions: An update. *Arterioscler. Thromb. Vasc. Biol.* 2000; 20:177-178.

[13] Muller JE, Tofler GH: Triggering and hourly variation of onset of arterial thrombosis. *Ann. Epidemiol.* 1992; 2:393-405

[14] Libby P: Current concepts of the pathogenesis of the acute coronary syndromes. *Circulation* 2001; 104:365-372.

[15] Davies MJ: The composition of coronary artery plaque. *N. Engl. J .Med.* 1997; 336:1312-13.

[16] Burke AP, Farb A, Malcolm GT, et al: Coronary risk factors and plaque morphology in men with coronary disease who died suddenly. *N. Engl. J. med.* 1997; 336:1276-1282

[17] Kwon HM, et al: Enhanced coronary vasa vasorum neovascularization in experimental hypercholesterolemia. *J. Clin. Invest.* 1998; 101:1551-1556

[18] Assoian RK, Marcantonio EE: The extracellular matrix as a cell cycle control element in atherosclerosis and restenosis. *J. Clin. Invest.* 1996; 98:2436-2439

[19] Davies MJ, Gordon JL, Gearing AJ, et al: The expression of the adhesion molecules ICAM-1, VCAM-1, PECAM, and E- selectin in human atherosclerosis. *J. Pathol.* 1993; 171:223-229

[20] Massberg S, Brand K, Gruner S, et al: A critical role of platelet adhesion in the initiation of atherosclerotic lesion formation. *J. Exp. Med.* 2002;196:887-896.

[21] Kroll M, Sullivan R: Mechanisms of platelet activation, in Loscalzo JA, Schafer A [eds]: Thrombosis and Haemorrhage. Philadelphia PA, Williams and Wilkins, 1998;261-291.

[22] Lefcovits J, Plow EF, Topol EJ: Platelet glycoprotein IIb/IIIa receptors in cardiovascular medicine. *N .Engl .J. Med* .1995;332:1553-1559

[23] Arbustini EDBB, Morbini P, Burke AP, Bocciarelli M, Specchia G, Virmani: Plaque erosion is a major substrate for coronary thrombosis in acute myocardial infarction. *Heart* 1999; 82:269-72

[24] Ross R. Atherosclerosis - An Inflammatory Disease. *Atherosclerosis.* 1999; 340:115-126.

[25] Falk e. Pathogenesis of atherosclerosis. *J. Am. Coll. Cardiol.* 2006;47:7-12

[26] Libby P, Theroux P: Pathophysiology of Coronary Artery Disease. *Circulation* 2005;111:3481-3488.

[27] Smith S, Blair S, Bonow R, et al: AHA/ACC Guidelines for Preventing Heart Attack and Death in Patients With Atherosclerotic Cardiovascular Disease: 2001 Update. *Circulation* 2001;104: 1577-1579.

[28] Ambrosioni E, Bacchelli S, Esposti DD, Borghi C:Anti-ischemic effects of angiotensin-converting enzyme inhibitors: a future therapeutic perspective. *J. Cardiovasc. Pharmacol.* 2001;37 [Suppl 1]:S3-9.

[29] Curzen NP, Fox KM: Do ACE inhibitors modulate atherosclerosis?. *Eur. Heart J.* 1997;18[10]:1530-5.

[30] Wannamethee S, Lowe G, Shaper A et al: The metabolic syndrome and insulin resistance: relationship to haemostatic and inflammatory markers in older non-diabetic men. *Atherosclerosis.* 2005; 181[1]:101-108.

[31] Pedersen, T.R., L.Wilhelmsen, O.Faergeman, et al.: Follow-up study of patients randomized in the Scandinavian Simvastatin Survival Study [4S] of cholesterol lowering. *Am. J. Cardiol.* 2000;86:257-262

[32] Ascer E, Bertolami M, Venturinelli M et al: Atorvastatin reduces proinflammatory markers in hypercholesterolemic patients. *Atherosclerosis.* 2004; Vol.177 [1]: 161-166

[33] Yusuf S. Clopidogrel in unstable angina to prevent recurrent ischemic events [CURE]. Program and abstracts of the American College of Cardiology 50-th Annual Scientific Session; March 18-21,2001;Orlando Florida, Presentation 9, Session 405.

[34] EPILOG Investigators. Platelet glycoprotein IIb/IIa receptor blockade and low-dose heparin during percutaneous coronary revascularization. *N. Engl. J. Med.* 1997;336:1689-96.

Index

D

E

F

G

N

O

P

Q

R

S

T

U

V

W